CHAIR YOGA FOR SENIORS OVER 60

TRANSFORMATIVE YOGA PRACTICES FOR MIND, BODY, AND SOUL

HARMONY VOYAGER

Contents

Introduction

Welcome to "Seat Yoga for Seniors: <u>Embrace Your Health Process After 60</u>."

As we age, keeping up with actual wellbeing and mental prosperity turns out to be progressively significant. This book is planned explicitly for seniors who try to upgrade their personal satisfaction through delicate, available yoga rehearses. Whether you are new to yoga or hoping to adjust your current practice, seat yoga offers a protected and viable method for remaining dynamic and associated with your body.

Seat yoga gives every one of the advantages of customary yoga, including further developed adaptability, strength, and equilibrium, while involving a seat for help. This makes it an ideal choice for the people who could find floor-based practices testing. The developments are basic yet compelling, zeroing in on breathing methods, extending, and unwinding, which are crucial for keeping up with wellbeing and essentialness.

Our process together will investigate different postures and schedules custom fitted to address the issues of seniors. Every section offers definite guidelines, changes, and tips to guarantee you can rehearse securely and unhesitatingly. Furthermore, you will track down direction on establishing a serene practice climate, laying out reasonable objectives, and paying attention to your body.

Integrating seat yoga into your day to day schedule can prompt various advantages, like lessening pressure, expanding course, and improving mental lucidity. It likewise furnishes a brilliant chance to interface with yourself, cultivating a feeling of harmony and prosperity.

Keep in mind, it's never beyond any good time to begin a novel, new thing. Seat yoga welcomes you to find a delicate way to wellbeing and satisfaction. How about we set out on this excursion together, embracing every second with beauty and appreciation. Welcome to a lively, enabled section of your life.

.

What You Need to Know Before Getting Started

Leaving on your seat yoga venture is an interesting step towards improving your prosperity. The following are a couple of significant things to remember before you start:

1. Counsel Your Medical care Supplier

Prior to beginning any new activity program, it's fundamental for check with your PCP, particularly in the event that you have any current ailments or concerns. Your medical services supplier can offer customized guidance and guarantee that seat yoga is a protected choice for you.

2. Pick the Right Seat

Select a tough, stable seat without wheels. A seat with a straight back and no armrests is great, as it considers a full scope of movement. Guarantee the seat is put on a non-slip surface to keep it from moving during your training.

3. Wear Open to Attire

Choose free, happy with apparel that permits you to openly move. Keep away from tight or prohibitive articles of clothing that could hinder your developments or relaxing.

4. Set Up a Place of refuge

Make a quiet, mess free climate where you can zero in on your training. Guarantee you have sufficient room around you to expand your arms and legs without block. A peaceful, very much ventilated room is great for unwinding and fixation.

5. Assemble Vital Props

While seat yoga is open, having a couple of props close by can upgrade your training. Think about utilizing:

A little pad or collapsed cover for additional solace.

A yoga tie or a belt to help with extends.

Light loads or opposition groups for added strength preparing, whenever suggested by your medical services supplier.

6. Pay attention to Your Body

Give close consideration to how your body feels during each posture. It's generally expected to feel a delicate stretch, however you ought to never encounter torment or distress. In the event that a development doesn't feel right, change the posture or skip it through and through. Over the long haul, you'll turn out to be more sensitive to your body's signs and limits.

7. Begin Slow and Advance Steadily

In the event that you're new to yoga or haven't practiced in some time, begin with short meetings and continuously increment the length and force. Consistency is critical, and, surprisingly, a couple of moments daily can have a huge effect after some time.

8. Center around Your Breath

Breathing is a key part of yoga. Focus on your breath, taking sluggish, profound breathes in and breathes out. This supports your actual developments as well as advances unwinding and mental lucidity.

9. Remain Hydrated

Drink a lot of water when your training. Remaining hydrated keeps up with your energy levels and supports in general wellbeing.

10. Partake in the Excursion

Yoga isn't just about actual activity; an all encompassing practice sustains the body, psyche, and soul. Move toward every meeting with an open heart and brain, partaking all the while and commending your advancement, regardless of how little.

By remembering these focuses, you'll be completely ready to begin your seat yoga practice. Embrace this potential chance to improve your wellbeing and prosperity, each delicate stretch in turn.

What You Need to Know Before Getting Started

Leaving on your seat yoga adventure is an intriguing step towards working on your thriving. Coming up next are several critical things to recollect before you start:

1. Counsel Your Clinical consideration Provider

Before starting any new action program, it's key for check with your PCP, especially if you have any ongoing diseases or concerns. Your clinical benefits provider can offer tweaked direction and assurance that seat yoga is a safeguarded decision for you.

2. Pick the Right Seat

Select an extreme, stable seat without wheels. A seat with a straight back and no armrests is perfect, as it thinks about a full extent of development. Ensure the seat is placed on a non-slip surface to hold it back from moving during your preparation.

3. Wear Open to Clothing

Pick free, content with attire that licenses you to move transparently. Avoid tight or restrictive pieces of clothing that could frustrate your turns of events or unwinding.

4. Set Up a Safe space

Make a calm, wreck free environment where you can focus in on your preparation. Promise you have adequate space around you to extend your arms and legs without block. A quiet, a lot of ventilated room is perfect for loosening up and obsession.

5. Collect Imperative Props

While seat yoga is open, having several props nearby can update your preparation. Ponder using:

A little cushion or imploded cover for extra comfort.

A yoga tie or a belt to assist with broadens.

Light loads or resistance bunches for added strength getting ready, at whatever point recommended by your clinical benefits provider.

6. Focus on Your Body

Give close thought to how your body feels during each stance. It's for the most part expected to feel a fragile stretch, but you should never experience torture or trouble. If an improvement doesn't feel right, change the stance or skip it totally. Over an extended time, you'll end up being more delicate to your body's signs and cutoff points.

7. Start Slow and Progress Consistently

If you're new to yoga or haven't polished in some time, start with short gatherings and consistently increase the length and power. Consistency is basic, and, shockingly, several minutes everyday can have a gigantic impact after some time.

8. Base on Your Breath

Breathing is a critical piece of yoga. Center around your breath, taking slow, significant takes in and inhales out. This supports your genuine improvements as well as advances loosening up and mental clarity.

9. Stay Hydrated

Hydrate while your preparation. Staying hydrated stays aware of your energy levels and supports in everyday prosperity.

10. Participate in the Outing

Yoga isn't just about genuine movement; a sweeping practice supports the body, mind, and soul. Push toward each gathering with an open heart and cerebrum, sharing meanwhile and recognizing your progression, paying little mind to how little.

By recollecting these centers, you'll be totally prepared to start your seat yoga practice. Embrace this likely opportunity to work on your prosperity and thriving, every single fragile stretch.

What is Yoga and Its History

What is Yoga?

Yoga is a comprehensive practice that joins the body, psyche, and soul through actual stances (asanas), breath control (pranayama), and reflection (dhyana). Beginning from antiquated India, yoga expects to advance generally prosperity by improving adaptability, strength, balance, and mental clearness. "Yoga" is gotten from the Sanskrit root "yuj," signifying "to burden" or "to join together," representing the association of individual awareness with all inclusive cognizance.

Yoga includes different styles and works on, going from delicate and helpful to energetic and dynamic. No matter what the style, the embodiment of yoga lies in care, mindfulness, and internal harmony.

The Historical backdrop of Yoga

The historical backdrop of yoga is rich and complex, traversing millennia. Here is a short outline of its development:

Vedic Period (1500 - 500 BCE)

The earliest references to yoga are tracked down in the Vedas, antiquated holy texts of India. During this period, yoga was fundamentally a profound work on including customs, serenades, and contemplation to interface with the heavenly.

Pre-Traditional Period (500 BCE - 200 CE)

The Upanishads, philosophical texts that followed the Vedas, developed the profound parts of yoga, stressing contemplation and the internal excursion to self-acknowledgment.

The Bhagavad Gita, a holy sacred text from this period, presents the idea of yoga as a way to exemplary nature and obligation, consolidating different structures like Bhakti (commitment), Jnana (information), and Karma (activity).

Traditional Period (200 CE - 500 CE)

The traditional period is set apart by the organization of the Yoga Sutras of Patanjali, a basic text that arranged the act of yoga. Patanjali's eight-limbed way (Ashtanga) frames the phases of yoga practice: Yama (moral norms), Niyama (self-restraint), Asana (stances), Pranayama (breath control), Pratyahara (withdrawal of faculties), Dharana (fixation), Dhyana (contemplation), and Samadhi (illumination).

Post-Old style Period (500 CE - 1500 CE)

During this period, yoga aces grew new strategies to restore the body and delay life. This period saw the development of Hatha Yoga, zeroing in on actual stances and breath control to set up the body for more profound reflection.

Current Period (Late nineteenth 100 years - Present)

Yoga was acquainted with the Western world in the late nineteenth and mid twentieth hundreds of years by Indian yogis like Master Vivekananda and Paramahansa Yogananda. Their lessons accentuated the otherworldly and philosophical parts of yoga.

During the twentieth 100 years, figures like B.K.S. Iyengar, Pattabhi Jois, and Indra Devi promoted Hatha Yoga and its different styles, making it open to a worldwide crowd.

Today, yoga keeps on advancing, coordinating conventional practices with contemporary wellbeing and health patterns. It is generally perceived for its physical, mental, and otherworldly advantages, drawing in great many specialists around the world.

The Advantages of Yoga

Yoga offers a large number of advantages, including:

Further developed adaptability, strength, and equilibrium.
Upgraded respiratory capability and cardiovascular wellbeing.
Diminished pressure, tension, and discouragement.
Expanded mental lucidity and concentration.
Better rest and in general unwinding.
A more profound feeling of association and internal harmony.
Whether you are looking for actual wellness, stress help, or otherworldly development, yoga gives a flexible and all encompassing way to deal with working on your personal satisfaction. As you leave on this excursion, you'll find the immortal insight and significant advantages that yoga brings to the table.

Types of Yoga and Their Principles

Sorts of Yoga

Yoga wraps a considerable number styles and practices, each with its fascinating focus and benefits. Here are unquestionably the most notable sorts of yoga:

Hatha Yoga

Depiction: Habitually remembered to be the supporting of all yoga practices, Hatha Yoga bases on genuine positions (asanas) and breath control (pranayama).
Benefits: Further creates flexibility, strength, and harmony; propels loosening up and push help.

Vinyasa Yoga

Depiction: Known for its fluid, strong progressions that synchronize breath with improvement. As often as possible suggested as "stream" yoga.

Benefits: Overhauls cardiovascular prosperity, grows flexibility and strength, and gives an intelligent, melodic practice.

Ashtanga Yoga

Portrayal: An intensive, coordinated practice with a specific gathering of positions, associated by breath and improvement.

Benefits: Creates grit, flexibility, and perseverance; propels discipline and mental focus.

Iyengar Yoga

Portrayal: Stresses accurate game plan and the usage of props like blocks, lashes, and builds up to achieve the right position.

Benefits: Further creates plan, balance, and flexibility; sensible for all levels, integrating those with real cutoff points.

Bikram Yoga

Depiction: Contains a set progression of 26 positions practiced in a warmed room (around 105°F or 40°C) to propel detoxification and flexibility.

Benefits: Further develops flexibility, strength, and constancy; maintains detoxification through sweating.

Kundalini Yoga

Depiction: Joins genuine positions, breath exercises, recounting, and reflection to mix the kundalini energy at the groundwork of the spine.

Benefits: Redesigns significant care, near and dear harmony, and genuine vitality.

Yin Yoga

Depiction: A drowsy paced style where stances are held for a couple of moments to target significant connective tissues and advance loosening up.

Benefits: Additions flexibility, deals with joint prosperity, and instigates a mysterious legislature of loosening up.

Steady Yoga

Portrayal: Spotlights on loosening up and recovery, including props to help the body in loosening up stances.
Benefits: Diminishes pressure, progresses recovering, and balances the tangible framework.
Pre-birth Yoga

Portrayal: Uniquely crafted for pregnant women, focusing in on fragile broadening, breath work, and mental centering.
Benefits: Redesigns flexibility and strength, decreases pregnancy-related disquiet, and prepares the body and cerebrum for work.
Seat Yoga

Portrayal: Changes customary yoga positions to be performed arranged in a seat or including a seat for help.

Benefits: Grows flexibility, strength, and harmony; open for seniors and those with adaptability issues.

Norms of Yoga

Regardless of what the sort of yoga practiced, a couple of focus principles underlie the preparation:

Ahimsa (**Serenity**)

Advance toward your preparation and presence with mindfulness and compassion, avoiding wickedness to yourself as well as others.

Satya (Genuineness)

Embrace dependability and validity in your perspectives, words, and exercises.

Asteya (Non-taking)

Foster a sensation of joy and make an effort not to want what others have, whether it's material things or qualities.

Brahmacharya (Equilibrium)

Practice control in all pieces of life, changing needs and inspirations.

Aparigraha (Non-possessiveness)

Surrender association with resources and results, empowering a sensation of chance and fulfillment.

Saucha (Flawlessness)

Stay aware of tidiness in your body, mind, and environment, propelling prosperity and clarity.

Santosha (Bliss)

Foster a disposition of appreciation and fulfillment, enduring things as they are.

Tapas (Discipline)

Center around normal practice and self control, overcoming hindrances truly.

Svadhyaya (Self-study)

Partake in examination and relentless getting, attempting to fathom yourself better.

Ishvara Pranidhana (Surrender to a Higher Power)

See and regard a more powerful, surrendering private mental self portrait and embracing lowliness.

These principles, regularly suggested as the Yamas and Niyamas in the Yoga Sutras of Patanjali, give a moral and moral beginning stage for yoga work on, coordinating experts toward a good and genial life. By integrating these norms into your preparation and everyday presence, you can experience the full notable ability of yoga.

Advantages of Chair Yoga

Seat yoga is a sensitive sort of yoga practiced while sitting on a seat or including a seat for help. This open style of yoga offers different benefits, particularly for seniors, individuals with convenience issues, or those new to yoga. **The following are a couple of basic advantages of seat yoga:**

1. Further creates Versatility

Seat yoga helps increase versatility by carefully expanding muscles and joints. Standard practice can work on your extent of development, simplifying regular activities and more pleasant.

2. Overhauls Strength

By performing various stances and improvements, seat yoga creates and stay aware of muscle courage. This is particularly useful for seniors, as staying aware of mass is dire for in everyday prosperity and independence.

3. Upholds Balance and Coordination

Seat yoga consolidates rehearses that further foster balance and coordination, reducing the bet of falls. Redesigned balance is pivotal for staying aware of versatility and confidence in performing standard tasks.

4. Diminishes Strain and Anxiety

The accentuation on breath control and care in seat yoga propels loosening up and diminishes pressure. Practicing seat yoga can help with cutting down disquiet levels and redesign up close and personal flourishing.

5. Maintains Joint Prosperity

Fragile advancements in seat yoga help with lubing up the joints, reducing robustness and chipping away at joint prosperity. This is especially significant for individuals with joint agony or other joint-related conditions.

6. Grows Spread

Seat yoga propels better blood stream, which can chip away at overall cardiovascular prosperity and help with lessening results of relentless conditions like hypertension and diabetes.

7. Works on Respiratory Capacity

Breathing exercises (pranayama) united in seat yoga can additionally foster lung limit and respiratory adequacy. Better breathing techniques furthermore add to extended energy levels and loosening up.

8. Open to All Health Levels

Seat yoga is flexible and can be changed to suit different wellbeing levels and real limits. An astonishing decision for individuals could find standard yoga presents testing since mature enough, injury, or confined versatility.

9. Accommodating and Versatile

Seat yoga can be practiced wherever, settling on it a supportive decision for those with limited space or time. All you truly need is areas of strength for an and a little locale to practice.

10. Deals with Mental Clearness and Focus

The intelligent pieces of seat yoga help with sharpening mental clearness and further foster concentration. Standard practice can work on mental ability and add to better mental prosperity.

11. Propels Social Affiliation

Bundle seat yoga classes give an entryway to social collaboration, empowering a sensation of neighborhood diminishing impressions of withdrawal, which is particularly useful for seniors.

12. Maintains Torture The board

Seat yoga can be a sensitive technique for directing and decrease steady torture. The slow, cautious turns of events and stretches can relieve disquiet in areas like the back, neck, and shoulders.

13. Enables Care

Seat yoga stimulates care and body care. By focusing in on the ongoing second and communicating with your breath and improvements, you can foster a more imperative sensation of internal concordance and success.

Seat yoga is an adaptable and strong practice that offers a broad assortment of physical, mental, and significant benefits. Whether you are attempting to deal with your overall prosperity, manage a specific condition, or simply track down a fragile technique for staying dynamic, seat yoga can be a sublime extension to your wellbeing plan.

Key Focus points

Seat yoga is a delicate and open type of yoga that offers various advantages, especially for seniors and people with restricted portability. Here are the key focus points:

Further developed Adaptability and Strength

Seat yoga improves adaptability and muscle strength, supporting everyday exercises and advancing generally actual wellbeing.

Better Equilibrium and Coordination

Normal practice further develops equilibrium and coordination, diminishing the gamble of falls and upgrading versatility.

Stress and Uneasiness Decrease

The emphasis on breath control and care assists lower with focusing on and nervousness levels, adding to profound prosperity.

Joint Wellbeing and Flow

Delicate developments support joint wellbeing and further develop flow, helping those with joint pain or other persistent circumstances.

Improved Respiratory Capability

Breathing activities remembered for seat yoga further develop lung limit and respiratory productivity, helping generally energy levels.

Openness

Seat yoga is versatile to different wellness levels and actual capacities, making it appropriate for seniors, those recuperating from wounds, and novices.

Accommodation

Seat yoga can be drilled anyplace with negligible space and gear, offering a helpful method for integrating exercise into your day to day daily schedule.

Mental Clearness and Concentration

The thoughtful parts of seat yoga upgrade mental lucidity, focus, and mental capability.

Social Collaboration

Bunch seat yoga classes give potential open doors to social commitment, cultivating a feeling of local area and lessening sensations of seclusion.

Torment The board

Delicate stretches and careful developments in seat yoga can help oversee and ease constant agony.

Care and Inward Harmony

Seat yoga advances care and body mindfulness, adding to a more noteworthy feeling of inward harmony and in general prosperity.

Integrating seat yoga into your routine can prompt critical upgrades in actual wellbeing, mental clearness, and profound equilibrium. A flexible and viable practice upholds an all encompassing way to deal with health, settling on it a phenomenal decision for improving personal satisfaction.

How to Prepare Yourself for Yoga

Getting ready for a yoga meeting, particularly in the event that you're new to the training or participating in seat yoga, includes both physical and mental planning. Here are a moves toward assist you with preparing:

1. Counsel Your Medical care Supplier
Prior to beginning any new activity routine, particularly assuming you have previous ailments or concerns, counsel your primary care physician to guarantee that yoga is a protected and suitable action for you.

2. Pick the Right Gear
Seat: Select a strong, stable seat without wheels. A seat with a straight back and no armrests is great.
Yoga Mat: If utilizing a mat, guarantee it's put on a non-slip surface to forestall any development.

Props: Have strong props like pads, yoga blocks, lashes, or a collapsed cover close by to upgrade solace and backing during your training.

3. Wear Open to Dress

Choose free, happy with apparel that permits free development. Keep away from tight or prohibitive articles of clothing that could thwart your developments or relaxing.

4. Establish a Quiet Climate

Set up a tranquil, mess free space where you can zero in on your training without interruptions. A peaceful, very much ventilated room is great for unwinding and focus.

5. Remain Hydrated

Drink a lot of water when your yoga meeting. Remaining hydrated keeps up with your energy levels and supports in general wellbeing.

6. Eat Daintily

Try not to rehearse yoga after having just eaten a lot. Have a light bite or feast no less than 1-2 hours before your meeting to forestall uneasiness during presents.

7. Warm-Up

Start with delicate warm-up activities to set up your body for yoga. Straightforward stretches or developments can assist with releasing your muscles and joints, decreasing the gamble of injury.

8. Set Your Goal

Pause for a minute to set a positive goal for your training. This could be a particular objective, like further developing adaptability, or a general point, such as discovering a genuine sense of harmony.

9. Center around Your Breath

Begin by focusing on your breath. Profound, careful breathing aides community your brain and set up your body for the developments ahead.

10. Be Aware of Your Cutoff points

Pay attention to your body and regard its cutoff points. Abstain from propelling yourself excessively hard or endeavoring represents that cause agony or inconvenience. Adjust acts like required and steadily develop your training.

11. Accumulate Extra Assets

Consider utilizing yoga books, online recordings, or applications intended for seat yoga to direct your training. These assets can give accommodating guidelines, adjustments, and schedules fit to your necessities.

12. Practice Routinely

Consistency is critical to receiving the rewards of yoga. Mean to integrate yoga into your daily schedule consistently, regardless of whether it's only a couple of moments every day.

13. Remain Positive and Patient

Progress in yoga can take time. Remain positive, show restraint toward yourself, and celebrate little accomplishments en route.

By following these means, you'll be good to go to begin your yoga process. Seat yoga, specifically, offers a delicate and open method for further developing your physical and mental prosperity, making it a superb expansion to your day to day daily practice.

Building the Right Mentality for Yoga

A positive and open mentality is fundamental for a remunerating yoga practice. Here are a few vital methodologies to assist with developing the perfect mental disposition:

1. Embrace a Novice's Brain

Move toward every yoga meeting with interest and receptiveness, no matter what your experience level. Relinquish assumptions and learn and investigate.

2. Put forth Practical Objectives

Lay out reachable objectives for your training. Whether it's further developing adaptability, diminishing pressure, or discovering an authentic sense of harmony, having clear goals can inspire you and give guidance.

3. Be Available

Center around the current second. Yoga isn't just about actual postures yet in addition about associating with your breath and being aware of your body and considerations. Practice care and let go of interruptions.

4. Practice Self-Empathy

Be thoughtful to yourself. Recognize your impediments and commend your advancement, regardless of how little. Keep away from self-analysis and embrace a sustaining disposition towards your body and psyche.

5. Develop Tolerance

Comprehend that advancement in yoga is slow. Show restraint toward yourself and permit your training to advance normally after some time. Try not to rush or propelling yourself excessively hard.

6. Remain Positive

Keep an uplifting outlook. Center around the advantages of your training and how it affects you as opposed to contrasting yourself with others. Commend your endeavors and accomplishments.

7. Relinquish Assumptions

Discharge any assumptions regarding what your training "ought to" seem to be.

Every meeting is extraordinary, and it's critical to acknowledge and embrace where you are in your excursion.

8. Focus on Standard Practice

Consistency is critical to building areas of strength for a training. Devote an ordinary time for yoga, regardless of whether it's only a couple of moments every day. Customary pursue supports positive routines and outlook.

9. Center around the Breath

Utilize your breath as an anchor. Profound, careful breathing can assist with quieting the psyche, lessen pressure, and keep you centered during your training. Focus on your inward breaths and exhalations, utilizing them to direct your developments.

10. Acknowledge and Embrace Change

Perceive that both your body and psyche are continually evolving. What feels open one day may be testing the following. Embrace these changes as a feature of your yoga process.

11. Look for Motivation

Find motivation through yoga books, classes, recordings, or local gatherings. Gaining from others and sharing encounters can advance your training and assist you with remaining inspired.

12. Practice Appreciation

Develop a feeling of appreciation for your body, your training, and the time you devote to taking care of oneself. Appreciation can improve your general yoga experience and advance an uplifting perspective.

13. Interface with a Local area

Join a yoga class or gathering, either face to face or on the web. Being essential for a local area can offer help, support, and a feeling of having a place.

By embracing these procedures, you can fabricate an outlook that upholds a satisfying and supportable yoga practice. Keep in mind, yoga is an excursion of self-disclosure and development. Embrace it with an open heart and psyche, and partake in the many advantages it brings to your physical, mental, and close to home prosperity.

Your First Yoga Poses

Starting with simple and open yoga positions can help you build a lot of grit for your planning. Coming up next are two or three juvenile obliging situations to get you rolling, each with point by point explanations:

1. Coordinated Mountain Position (Tadasana)

Portrayal: This principal position helps you with spreading out certified position and system while sitting.

How to Get Things Moving:

Sit tranquilly on a seat with your feet level on the floor, hip-width isolated.

Keep your spine straight, bears free, and hands laying on your thighs.

Stretch your neck and imagine a string gently pulling the main trait of your head toward the rooftop.

Take in basically and stand firm on the footing for a few breaths, feeling grounded and centered.

2. Coordinated Ahead Bend (Paschimottanasana)

Depiction: a gentle stretch for the legs and back that improves flexibility and relaxation.

Things to do to get it going:

Sit on the edge of the seat with your feet level on the floor.

Take in and stretch your spine.

Take in out and bit by bit reshape forward from the hips, showing up at your hands towards your feet or the floor.

Let your head and neck unwind, and take in on a very basic level.

After a few deep breaths, slowly and incrementally return to an organized position.

3. Coordinated Cat Cow Stretch (Marjaryasana-Bitilasana)

Portrayal: This significant improvement contributes to the development of spine adaptability and further encourages action.

Headings to Get it moving:

With your hands down, sit on a seat.

Take in, contort your back, and move in the direction of the sky, allowing your stomach to drop towards the floor (Cow Position).

Take in out, round your spine, and overlay your jaw towards your chest (Cat Position).

For two or three cycles, alternate between the fetuses and cows.

4. Coordinated Spinal Bend (Ardha Matsyendrasana)

Portrayal: a breeze to control and take care of spinal adaptability.

To get it moving, it needs bearings:

Sit sideways on the seat with your right side defying the seat back.

Put your hands on the back of the seat.

Take in and stretch your spine.

Take in out and carefully bend your center aside, exploring your right shoulder.

Take a few deep breaths while you hold the breeze and then come back to the middle.

Repeat on the left side.

5. Coordinated Pigeon Position (Eka Pada Rajakapotasana)

Portrayal: Opens the hips and stretches the glutes and thighs.

Direction to Get it going:

Sit on the edge of the seat with your feet level on the floor.

Lift your right lower leg and place it over your knee on your left side thigh.

In order to shield your knee, flex your right foot.

To extend the stretch, sit tall and, if it feels good, lean slightly forward.

Stand firm on the footing for a couple of breaths, then, switch sides.

6. Coordinated Side Stretch (Parsva Tadasana)

Portrayal: Extends the sides of your body and further makes adaptability.

Each little move toward turn direction to Get it going:

Place your feet flat on the ground while seated in a seat.

Take in, stretch your spine, and raise your right arm in the air.

Cover your left side delicately as you breathe out and feel a stretch along your right side.

Get back to the center subsequent to holding the stretch for a couple of breaths.

Rehash truly side.

7. Illustration of Coordinated Knee-to-Chest (Apanasana):

a gentle stretch for the hips and lower back.

The most effective strategy is:

Put your feet level on the ground while situated in a seat.

Holding your right knee with two hands, raise it toward your chest.

Keep your back straight and shoulders free.

Stand firm on the traction for several breaths, then, transport and rehash with the left knee.

These positions are required to have been open and basic for youngsters, especially those rehearsing seat yoga. Attempt to move delicately, rotate around your body, and take in essentially all through each position. As you get more comfortable with these central positions, you can look at positions and groups that aren't made. You can even make a small turn.

Simple and Quick Standing and Floor-Based Yoga Postures

Here are a few fledgling accommodating standing and floor-based yoga represents that are not difficult to perform and give a fast, powerful practice:

Mountain Pose (Tadasana), a standing yoga pose, is described as follows: a fundamental pose that strengthens core stability and posture.

Step by step instructions to Make it happen:

With your feet hip-width apart, stand.

Disseminate your weight equally across the two feet.

Lift your kneecaps, engage your thighs, and lengthen your spine.

Loosen up your shoulders and let your arms hang by your sides.

Inhale profoundly and hold for a few breaths.

Tree Posture (Vrksasana)

Depiction: bolsters leg strength and improves balance.

Step by step instructions to Make it happen:

Stand with feet together.

Shift your weight onto your left foot and put your right foot to your left side internal thigh or calf (keep away from the knee).

Carry your hands to your heart community or above.

Hold for a few breaths, then switch sides.

Description of Warrior II (Virabhadrasana II): Reinforces the legs and arms, and opens the hips.

What to Do:

Stand with feet wide separated.

Put your left foot slightly in and your right foot 90 degrees out.

Make sure your right knee is bent over your ankle.

Stretch out your arms out to the sides, lined up with the floor.

Hold your gaze over your right hand for a few deep breaths.

Change sides.

Forward Crease (Uttanasana)

Portrayal: stretches the lower back and hamstrings.

Instructions to Make it happen:

With your feet hip-width apart, stand.

Lengthen your spine as you inhale.

Breathe out, pivot at the hips, and overlay forward.

Allow your hands to touch the shins, ankles, or floor.

Loosen up your head and neck, and hold for a few breaths.

Seat Posture (Utkatasana)

Portrayal: bolsters core and legs strength.

What to Do:

Stand with feet hip-width separated.

Breathe in, raise your arms above.

Breathe out, twist your knees, and lower your hips as though sitting once more into a seat.

Keep your weight in your heels and your chest lifted.

Hold for a few seconds.

Floor-Based Yoga Stances

Kid's Posture (Balasana)

Portrayal: a seated position that stretches the hips and back.

What to Do:

With your big toes touching and your knees apart, kneel on the floor.

Sit out of sorts and expand your arms forward, bringing your brow down to the mat.

Inhale profoundly and unwind.

Feline Cow Stretch (Marjaryasana-Bitilasana)

Depiction: Works on spinal adaptability and alleviates strain.

The most effective method to Make it happen:
Begin on all fours in a tabletop position.
Breathe in, curve your back, and lift your head and tailbone (Cow Posture).
In Cat Pose, round your spine, tuck your chin into your chest, and exhale.
Rehash for a few breaths.

Cobra Posture (Bhujangasana)

Depiction: opens the chest and strengthens the back.
Instructions to Make it happen:
Lie face down with your hands under your shoulders.
Breathe in, press into your hands, and lift your chest off the floor.
Get your elbows marginally twisted and your shoulders far from your ears.
Hold for a couple of breaths, then lower down.

Situated Ahead Twist (Paschimottanasana)

Depiction: stretches the lower back and hamstrings.

The most effective method to Make it happen:

With your legs out in front of you, sit down.

Breathe in, protract your spine.

Reach for your feet and hinge at the hips as you exhale.

Hold for a few breaths, keeping your spine long.

Description of Bridge Pose (Setu Bandhasana): Reinforces the back and glutes, and opens the chest.

Step by step instructions to Make it happen:

With your knees bent and feet hip-width apart, lie on your back.

Press into your feet and lift your hips towards the roof.

Intertwine your fingers under your back and press your arms into the floor.

Hold for a few breaths, then, at that point, lower down.

By integrating these standing and floor-based yoga presents into your daily schedule, you can partake in a balanced practice that further develops adaptability, strength, and unwinding. Keep in mind to take a deep breath and move slowly through each pose.

Things to Avoid When Doing Yoga

Despite the fact that yoga is generally safe and beneficial, there are some things to avoid in order to ensure a safe and effective experience, particularly for seniors and beginners. The following are an essential things to avoid:

1. Make an effort not to Extend Past Your Limits

Why: Pushing too hard can incite wounds and disquiet.

What to Do In light of everything: Take note of your body's boundaries and pay attention to them. Start slowly and gradually increase the intensity as your flexibility and strength improve.

2. Try not to stop breathing for these reasons:

Pausing to breathe can increase pressure and reduce the training's benefits.

All things considered, what to do: Revolve around significant, reliable breathing all through your preparation. Use your breath to coordinate your turns of events and help you with loosening up.

3. Avoid comparing yourself to others. Why:

Each individual's body and practice are surprising, and assessments can incite dissatisfaction and weakness.

What to Do Taking everything into account: Commend your achievements, regardless of how little, and focus on your own advancement.

4. Do whatever it takes not to Perform Positions Erroneously

Why: An incorrect arrangement can result in harm and strain.

What to Do If all else fails: Center around authentic construction and game plan. If you are unsure, seek guidance from an experienced instructor or dependable resources to learn the appropriate methods.

5. Reasons Not to Practice With a Full Stomach:

Practicing yoga in the wake of having recently eaten a lot can cause trouble and upset improvement.

What to Do Taking everything into account: Wait at least one to two hours after eating before starting yoga. If vital, have a light snack before your gathering.

6. Try not to overwork yourself. Overstretching can lead to injuries to the joints and muscles.

What to Do in Its Place: Always and tenderly stretch. Never force your body into a position. To assist you with holding presents, use props like lashes or yoga blocks.

7. Keep the Warm-Up and Chill-Off in Mind:

Avoiding warm-up can provoke wounds, and excusing cool-down can cause muscle robustness.

What to Do If all else fails: Always begin with a gentle warm-up to acclimate your muscles and joints. Do a cool-down at the end of your workout to help your body and mind relax.

8. Avoid prolonged static poses because:

Holding models for quite a while can cause muscle weariness and burden, especially for fledglings.

What to Do in Its Place: Starting with more limited spans, progressively increment as strength and perseverance are created.

9. Do whatever it takes not to Practice Without Proper Equipment

Why: Using unseemly or lacking stuff can impact your security and prosperity.

What to Do Taking everything into account: Use a respectable quality yoga mat and consistent props like blocks, lashes, and builds up to redesign your preparation.

10. Why Not Overlook Torment?

A sign that something is wrong is pain, and ignoring it can exacerbate the issue.

What to Do Taking everything into account: If you experience pain, gently release yourself from the position. Change it until you find a pose or position that works for you.

11. Try not to practice in a dangerous environment:

Mishaps can happen while rehearsing in a dangerous or jumbled climate.

What to Do If all else fails: Verify that the outer layer of your training is non-slip, open, and clean. Dispose of any expected risks.

12. Reasons to Avoid Improper Clothes:

Clothing that is too close or prohibitive can make it hard to move and relax.

What to Do Taking everything into account: Wear pleasing, loose dress that grants free turn of events and genuine ventilation.

13. Avoid Neglecting Ailments for the Reasons:

Certain conditions may necessitate specific stance modifications or evasion.

What to Do About It: Prior to starting yoga, particularly assuming you have any worries or ailments, converse with your primary care physician. Follow a specific ideas or limitations they give.

By monitoring these careful steps and practices to avoid, you can ensure a safeguarded, enchanting, and effective yoga experience. Consistently center around your success and advance toward your preparation with care and respect for your body's necessities.

Yoga Routines for the Morning, Midday, and Evening

To assist you with beginning a solid and useful yoga practice, the morning, noontime, and evening meetings incorporate the accompanying tweaked schedules. Every ordinary splendid lights on various focuses to suit the hour of day and your necessities.

Morning yoga is a powerful technique for setting up your body and mind for the day and set a positive perspective. Base on addresses that vivify and expand your muscles.

Begin in Young person's Posture (Balasana) to zero in on the job that needs to be done and lay out a timetable for the day.

Hold for one to two minutes with significant unwinding.

Move to every one of the four situations for the catlike cow stretch (Marjaryasana-Bitilasana) for the catlike cow expands.

Keep your breath in a state of harmony with the progressions as you go through five to ten rounds.

Diving Confronting Canine (Adho Mukha Svanasana)

From the fours as a whole, lift your hips to Plunging Canine.

Hold for one to two minutes while accelerating your feet to extend your calves.

Legend I (Virabhadrasana I): On each side, step forward into Legend I.

Hold each side for 30 seconds to 1 second.

Uttanasana, or Remaining Forward Twist, includes collapsing forward from a situated position.

Loosen up your shoulders and neck by holding for one to two minutes.

Tadasana, or Mountain Posture, is: While in Mountain Posture, stand tall and focus on your breath and arrangement.
Hold for 1-2 minutes, feeling grounded and empowered.

Mid day

Plan for Early afternoon Yoga Enjoying some time off from your morning schedule to rehearse yoga around early afternoon can assist with restoring your brain and lighten any pressure that might have come about because of those exercises. This standard splendid lights on touchy widening and recharging.

Start with an arranged ahead contort (Paschimottanasana) to expand your back and hamstrings.
Hold for one to two minutes while profoundly relaxing.
Organized Turn (Ardha Matsyendrasana)

Play out an organized spinal turn on each side.

Hold one side for one to two minutes.
Feline Cow Stretch (Marjaryasana-Bitilasana)

Go over Feline Cow stretches to gather your spine.
Do five to ten rounds.
Range Position (Setu Bandhasana)

Lie on your back and lift into Stage Position.
Base on your breath as you hold for one to two minutes.
Benefits the-Wall Position (Viparita Karani)

Track down a wall and raise your legs.
To completely unwind and recharge, hold for five to ten minutes.

Evening Yoga Schedule

Evening yoga assists with relaxing your day, loosen up your body, and plan for peaceful rest. Zero in on addresses that help you relax and give up strain.

Youth's Position (Balasana)

Begin in Adolescent's Position to quiet your frontal cortex and body.

Hold for a few minutes while profoundly relaxing.

Act acknowledged like Reclining Bound Point Stance (Supta Baddha Konasana): Lay on your back with your feet together and your knees separated.

Hold for 2-3 minutes, loosening up your hips.

Arranged Ahead Bend (Paschimottanasana): To extend and slacken your back, play out an arranged ahead bend.

Hold for a few minutes while gradually relaxing.

(Supta Matsyendrasana) Prostrate Turn: Gradually contort your legs aside and afterward the other while lying on your back.

Hold each side for 2-3 minutes.

Benefits the-Wall Position (Viparita
Karani)

Lift your legs against a wall.
Hold for 5-10 minutes, zeroing in on
critical, quieting breaths.
Body Stance (Savasana): Finish in
Cadaver Posture for complete unwinding.
Lie level on your back with your palms
looking up, arms at your sides.
Give your body a full rest by holding for 5
to 10 minutes.
By integrating these schedules into your
day to day plan, you can receive the
rewards of yoga at different times over
the course of the day. This will help you
with staying empowered, focused, and
free. Focus on your body and make any
important acclimations to the postures
and spans.

Breathing Activities for Yoga

Breathing exercises, or pranayama, are an essential piece of yoga practice. They help to calm the mind, further foster fixation, and work on in everyday flourishing. The following are a couple of convincing breathing exercises sensible for youngsters and undeniable level specialists the equivalent:

1. Diaphragmatic Breathing (Stomach Unwinding)

Depiction: This focal breathing action helps you with attracting your stomach, progressing significant and useful unwinding.

Bit by bit directions to Get it going:

Sit or rests in a pleasing position.
Put one hand on your chest and the other on your midriff.
Take in significantly through your nose, allowing your waist to climb as it loads up

with air. Your chest should remain fairly still.

Inhale out comfortable through your nose or mouth, permitting your mid-area to fall.

Reiterate for 5-10 minutes, focusing in on the climb and fall of your waist.

2. Ujjayi Breathing (Effective Breath)

Portrayal: Much of the time used in Vinyasa and Ashtanga yoga, Ujjayi breathing makes a sensitive, oceanic sound and helps with synchronizing breath with improvement.

Bit by bit guidelines to Get it going:

Sit calmly with your spine straight.

Take in significantly through your nose, to some degree fixing the back of your throat like preliminaries up a mirror.

Inhale out through your nose, staying aware of the stifling in your throat to convey a sensitive mumbling sound.

Happen for 5-10 minutes, keeping a steady and even breath.

3. Nadi Shodhana (Substitute Nostril Unwinding)

Portrayal: This changing breath strategy helps with calming the mind and balance the tactile framework.

The best strategy to Get it going:

Sit effectively with your spine straight.
Use your right thumb to close your right nostril.
Take in comfortable and significantly through your left nostril.
Close your left nostril with your right ring finger, and conveyance your right nostril.
Inhale out relaxed and absolutely through your right nostril.
Take in through your right nostril, then close it with your right thumb.
Release your left nostril and inhale out through it.

Reiterate for 5-10 minutes, turning nostrils with each breath.

4. Kapalabhati (Skull Shimmering Breath)

Depiction: This invigorating breathing system incorporates strong exhalations and uninvolved internal breaths, cleansing the respiratory structure and energizing the body.

The best strategy to Get it going:

Sit effectively with your spine straight.
Take a significant take in through your nose.
Inhale out unequivocally through your nose, getting your stomach muscles with each exhalation. The internal breath will happen typically and inertly.
Perform 20-30 speedy breaths, then, take a significant take in and inhale out relaxed.
Go over for 2-3 rounds.
5. 4-7-8 Unwinding

Depiction: This relaxing breathing method is exceptional for decreasing pressure and propelling rest.

Bit by bit guidelines to Get it going:

Sit or rests peacefully.
Close your eyes and take in cautiously through your nose for a count of 4.
Stop your relaxing for a count of 7.
Inhale out absolutely through your mouth, making a whoosh sound, for a count of 8.
Go over for 4-8 cycles, focusing in on keeping a peaceful and reliable rhythm.
6. Bhramari (Bumble bee Breath)
Depiction: This calming breathing methodology incorporates uttering a mumbling sound, which helps with moderating the tangible framework and decline pressure.

The best strategy to Get it going:

Sit effectively with your spine straight.
Close your eyes and take a significant take in through your nose.
As you inhale out, make a low mumbling sound like a bumble bee, keeping your mouth shut.
Revolve around the vibration of the sound.
Repeat for 5-10 minutes, keeping a sensitive and reliable mumble.
7. Box Breathing (Square Unwinding)
Portrayal: This strategy helps with calming the mind and further develop concentrate, for the most part used truth be told and stress decline practices.

The best technique to Get it going:

Sit effectively with your spine straight.
Take in through your nose for a count of 4.
Stop your relaxing for a count of 4.

Inhale out through your nose for a count of 4.

Stop your relaxing for a count of 4.

Go over for 5-10 minutes, imagining a square with each breath.

By incorporating these breathing exercises into your regular day to day timetable or yoga practice, you can overhaul your overall thriving, diminish strain, and work on your focus and energy levels. Make a point to practice these techniques cautiously and gently, allowing your breath to stream regularly and calmly.

One-Week Beginner Yoga Program

This one-week yoga program is intended for fledglings, offering a fair blend of morning, noontime, and evening practices to assist you with building a predictable daily schedule. Every meeting centers around various parts of yoga, including extending, reinforcing, unwinding, and breathwork.

Day 1: Establishment and Breath

Morning: Empowering Stream (20 minutes)

Kid's Posture (Balasana) - 2 minutes
Feline Cow Stretch (Marjaryasana-Bitilasana) - 5 rounds
Descending Confronting Canine (Adho Mukha Svanasana) - 1 moment
Hero I (Virabhadrasana I) - 1 moment each side
Mountain Posture (Tadasana) - 2 minutes
Noontime: Unwind and Invigorate (10 minutes)

Situated Ahead Twist (Paschimottanasana) - 2 minutes
Situated Curve (Ardha Matsyendrasana) - 1 moment each side
Advantages the-Wall Posture (Viparita Karani) - 5 minutes
Evening: Unwinding (15 minutes)

Kid's Posture (Balasana) - 2 minutes
Recumbent Wind (Supta Matsyendrasana) - 2 minutes each side
Carcass Posture (Savasana) - 5 minutes
Day 2: Strength and Solidness
Morning: Reinforcing Stream (20 minutes)

Feline Cow Stretch (Marjaryasana-Bitilasana) - 5 rounds
Descending Confronting Canine (Adho Mukha Svanasana) - 1 moment
Hero II (Virabhadrasana II) - 1 moment each side
Seat Posture (Utkatasana) - 1 moment

Mountain Posture (Tadasana) - 2 minutes
Late morning: Early afternoon Stretch (10 minutes)

Situated Ahead Twist (Paschimottanasana) - 2 minutes
Span Posture (Setu Bandhasana) - 2 minutes
Advantages the-Wall Posture (Viparita Karani) - 5 minutes
Evening: Delicate Yoga (15 minutes)

Youngster's Posture (Balasana) - 2 minutes
Situated Ahead Twist (Paschimottanasana) - 2 minutes
Cadaver Posture (Savasana) - 5 minutes
Day 3: Adaptability and Equilibrium
Morning: Adaptability Stream (20 minutes)

Descending Confronting Canine (Adho Mukha Svanasana) - 1 moment

Tree Posture (Vrksasana) - 1 moment each side

Champion I (Virabhadrasana I) - 1 moment each side

Situated Ahead Curve (Paschimottanasana) - 2 minutes

Mountain Posture (Tadasana) - 2 minutes

Noontime: Unwind and Revive (10 minutes)

Situated Contort (Ardha Matsyendrasana) - 1 moment each side

Feline Cow Stretch (Marjaryasana-Bitilasana) - 5 rounds

Advantages the-Wall Posture (Viparita Karani) - 5 minutes

Evening: Night Unwinding (15 minutes)

Youngster's Posture (Balasana) - 2 minutes

Recumbent Wind (Supta Matsyendrasana) - 2 minutes each side

Carcass Posture (Savasana) - 5 minutes

Day 4: Center and Breath
Morning: Center Strength (20 minutes)

Feline Cow Stretch (Marjaryasana-Bitilasana) - 5 rounds
Descending Confronting Canine (Adho Mukha Svanasana) - 1 moment
Board Posture (Phalakasana) - 1 moment
Span Posture (Setu Bandhasana) - 2 minutes
Mountain Posture (Tadasana) - 2 minutes
Noontime: Invigorating Break (10 minutes)

Situated Ahead Curve (Paschimottanasana) - 2 minutes
Situated Wind (Ardha Matsyendrasana) - 1 moment each side
Advantages the-Wall Posture (Viparita Karani) - 5 minutes
Evening: Quieting Yoga (15 minutes)

Kid's Posture (Balasana) - 2 minutes

Leaning back Bound Point Posture (Supta Baddha Konasana) - 2 minutes
Body Posture (Savasana) - 5 minutes
Day 5: Full Body Stream
Morning: Full Body Stream (20 minutes)

Descending Confronting Canine (Adho Mukha Svanasana) - 1 moment
Champion II (Virabhadrasana II) - 1 moment each side
Tree Posture (Vrksasana) - 1 moment each side
Situated Ahead Curve (Paschimottanasana) - 2 minutes
Mountain Posture (Tadasana) - 2 minutes
Noontime: Fast Stretch (10 minutes)

Situated Contort (Ardha Matsyendrasana) - 1 moment each side
Feline Cow Stretch (Marjaryasana-Bitilasana) - 5 rounds
Advantages the-Wall Posture (Viparita Karani) - 5 minutes
Evening: Delicate Stretch (15 minutes)

Youngster's Posture (Balasana) - 2 minutes
Recumbent Wind (Supta Matsyendrasana) - 2 minutes each side
Carcass Posture (Savasana) - 5 minutes
Day 6: Equilibrium and Unwinding
Morning: Equilibrium and Strength (20 minutes)

Feline Cow Stretch (Marjaryasana-Bitilasana) - 5 rounds
Descending Confronting Canine (Adho Mukha Svanasana) - 1 moment
Tree Posture (Vrksasana) - 1 moment each side
Champion I (Virabhadrasana I) - 1 moment each side
Mountain Posture (Tadasana) - 2 minutes
Noontime: Early afternoon Re-energize (10 minutes)

Situated Ahead Twist (Paschimottanasana) - 2 minutes

Span Posture (Setu Bandhasana) - 2 minutes

Advantages the-Wall Posture (Viparita Karani) - 5 minutes

Evening: Profound Unwinding (15 minutes)

Youngster's Posture (Balasana) - 2 minutes

Leaning back Bound Point Posture (Supta Baddha Konasana) - 2 minutes

Body Posture (Savasana) - 5 minutes

Day 7: Delicate and Helpful

Morning: Delicate Stream (20 minutes)

Kid's Posture (Balasana) - 2 minutes

Feline Cow Stretch (Marjaryasana-Bitilasana) - 5 rounds

Descending Confronting Canine (Adho Mukha Svanasana) - 1 moment

Situated Ahead Curve (Paschimottanasana) - 2 minutes

Mountain Posture (Tadasana) - 2 minutes

Noontime: Unwind and Revive (10 minutes)

Situated Curve (Ardha Matsyendrasana) - 1 moment each side
Feline Cow Stretch (Marjaryasana-Bitilasana) - 5 rounds
Advantages the-Wall Posture (Viparita Karani) - 5 minutes
Evening: Complete Unwinding (15 minutes)

Youngster's Posture (Balasana) - 2 minutes
Recumbent Wind (Supta Matsyendrasana) - 2 minutes each side
Carcass Posture (Savasana) - 5 minutes
Tips for Progress:
Consistency: Attempt to rehearse at similar times every day to fabricate a daily schedule.
Stand by listening to Your Body: Regard your cutoff points and try not to drive into torment.

Inhale Profoundly: Spotlight on your breath, utilizing it to guide and support your developments.

Remain Hydrated: Hydrate when your training.

Use Props: Make sure to blocks, lashes, or pads to help your postures.

By following this one-week yoga program, you'll lay out serious areas of strength for a for your training, work on your adaptability and strength, and develop a feeling of quiet and unwinding over the course of your day.

Advanced 8 to 14 Day Yoga Program

This best in class yoga program is intended for specialists who have a strong groundwork and are hoping to develop their training. It integrates a blend of testing presents, high level procedures, and an emphasis on breathwork and contemplation. Every day incorporates morning, early afternoon, and night meetings, with expanding intricacy and force.

Day 8: Strength and Adaptability
Morning: Power Stream (30 minutes)

Sun Welcome (Surya Namaskar) - 5 rounds
Hero III (Virabhadrasana III) - 1 moment each side
Crow Posture (Bakasana) - 1 moment
Side Board (Vasisthasana) - 1 moment each side

Wild Thing (Camatkarasana) - 1 moment each side

Late morning: Hip Openers (20 minutes)

Pigeon Posture (Eka Pada Rajakapotasana) - 2 minutes each side

Reptile Posture (Utthan Pristhasana) - 2 minutes each side

Fire Log Posture (Agnistambhasana) - 2 minutes each side

Butterfly Posture (Baddha Konasana) - 3 minutes

Evening: Profound Stretch (20 minutes)

Leaning back Bound Point Posture (Supta Baddha Konasana) - 3 minutes

Recumbent Wind (Supta Matsyendrasana) - 2 minutes each side

Cheerful Child Posture (Ananda Balasana) - 3 minutes

Body Posture (Savasana) - 5 minutes

Day 9: Reversals and Equilibrium

Morning: Reversal Practice (30 minutes)

Dolphin Posture (Ardha Pincha Mayurasana) - 3 minutes
Headstand (Sirsasana) - 3 minutes
Lower arm Stand (Pincha Mayurasana) - 3 minutes
Handstand (Adho Mukha Vrksasana) - 3 minutes
Kid's Posture (Balasana) - 2 minutes
Late morning: Center Strength (20 minutes)

Boat Posture (Navasana) - 2 minutes
Side Board (Vasisthasana) - 1 moment each side
Board Posture (Phalakasana) - 2 minutes
Insect Posture (Salabhasana) - 2 minutes
Span Posture (Setu Bandhasana) - 3 minutes
Evening: Unwinding (20 minutes)

Kid's Posture (Balasana) - 3 minutes

Leaning back Hand-to-Huge Toe Posture (Supta Padangusthasana) - 2 minutes each side

Advantages the-Wall Posture (Viparita Karani) - 5 minutes

Carcass Posture (Savasana) - 5 minutes

Day 10: Backbends and Heart Openers

Morning: Heart Opening Stream (30 minutes)

Sun Welcome (Surya Namaskar) - 5 rounds

Camel Posture (Ustrasana) - 2 minutes

Wheel Posture (Urdhva Dhanurasana) - 2 minutes

Bow Posture (Dhanurasana) - 2 minutes

Fish Posture (Matsyasana) - 2 minutes

Late morning: Spinal Versatility (20 minutes)

Feline Cow Stretch (Marjaryasana-Bitilasana) - 5 rounds

Situated Turn (Ardha Matsyendrasana) - 2 minutes each side

String the Needle Posture (Parsva Balasana) - 2 minutes each side
Span Posture (Setu Bandhasana) - 3 minutes
Evening: Helpful Yoga (20 minutes)

Kid's Posture (Balasana) - 3 minutes
Leaning back Bound Point Posture (Supta Baddha Konasana) - 3 minutes
Prostrate Wind (Supta Matsyendrasana) - 2 minutes each side
Cadaver Posture (Savasana) - 5 minutes
Day 11: Full Body Joining
Morning: Dynamic Stream (30 minutes)

Sun Greetings (Surya Namaskar) - 5 rounds
Champion II (Virabhadrasana II) - 1 moment each side
Triangle Posture (Trikonasana) - 1 moment each side
Broadened Side Point Posture (Utthita Parsvakonasana) - 1 moment each side

Half Moon Posture (Ardha Chandrasana) - 1 moment each side
Late morning: Arm Adjusts (20 minutes)

Crow Posture (Bakasana) - 2 minutes
Eight-Point Posture (Astavakrasana) - 2 minutes each side
Firefly Posture (Tittibhasana) - 2 minutes
Side Crow Posture (Parsva Bakasana) - 2 minutes each side
Evening: Profound Stretch (20 minutes)

Leaning back Bound Point Posture (Supta Baddha Konasana) - 3 minutes
Recumbent Contort (Supta Matsyendrasana) - 2 minutes each side
Blissful Child Posture (Ananda Balasana) - 3 minutes
Cadaver Posture (Savasana) - 5 minutes

Day 12: High level Postures and Contemplation

Morning: High level Stream (30 minutes)

Sun Greetings (Surya Namaskar) - 5 rounds

Fighter III (Virabhadrasana III) - 1 moment each side

Ruler Artist Posture (Natarajasana) - 1 moment each side

Full Parts (Hanumanasana) - 2 minutes each side

Wheel Posture (Urdhva Dhanurasana) - 2 minutes

Noontime: Contemplation and Pranayama (20 minutes)

Substitute Nostril Breathing (Nadi Shodhana) - 5 minutes

Kapalabhati (Skull Sparkling Breath) - 3 minutes

Situated Contemplation - 10 minutes

Evening: Delicate Yoga (20 minutes)

Kid's Posture (Balasana) - 3 minutes
Situated Ahead Curve (Paschimottanasana) - 3 minutes
Prostrate Contort (Supta Matsyendrasana) - 2 minutes each side
Cadaver Posture (Savasana) - 5 minutes
Day 13: Equilibrium and Concentration
Morning: Equilibrium Stream (30 minutes)

Sun Welcome (Surya Namaskar) - 5 rounds
Tree Posture (Vrksasana) - 1 moment each side
Falcon Posture (Garudasana) - 1 moment each side
Hero III (Virabhadrasana III) - 1 moment each side
Half Moon Posture (Ardha Chandrasana) - 1 moment each side
Noontime: Center and Soundness (20 minutes)

Boat Posture (Navasana) - 2 minutes

Board Posture (Phalakasana) - 2 minutes
Side Board (Vasisthasana) - 1 moment each side
Beetle Posture (Salabhasana) - 2 minutes
Span Posture (Setu Bandhasana) - 3 minutes
Evening: Supportive Yoga (20 minutes)

Youngster's Posture (Balasana) - 3 minutes
Leaning back Bound Point Posture (Supta Baddha Konasana) - 3 minutes
Recumbent Contort (Supta Matsyendrasana) - 2 minutes each side
Cadaver Posture (Savasana) - 5 minutes
Day 14: Joining and Reflection
Morning: Full Body Stream (30 minutes)

Sun Welcome (Surya Namaskar) - 5 rounds
Fighter II (Virabhadrasana II) - 1 moment each side
Triangle Posture (Trikonasana) - 1 moment each side

Broadened Side Point Posture (Utthita Parsvakonasana) - 1 moment each side
Half Moon Posture (Ardha Chandrasana) - 1 moment each side
Noontime: High level Postures (20 minutes)

Crow Posture (Bakasana) - 2 minutes
Eight-Point Posture (Astavakrasana) - 2 minutes each side
Firefly Posture (Tittibhasana) - 2 minutes
Side Crow Posture (Parsva Bakasana) - 2 minutes each side
Evening: Reflection and Contemplation (20 minutes)

Situated Ahead Twist (Paschimottanasana) - 3 minutes
Recumbent Turn (Supta Matsyendrasana) - 2 minutes each side
Situated Reflection - 10 minutes
Carcass Posture (Savasana) - 5 minutes
Tips for Cutting edge Professionals:

Warm-Up Appropriately: Guarantee an intensive get ready to set up your body for cutting edge presents.

Center around Arrangement: Appropriate arrangement is essential to forestall wounds.

Use Props: Use blocks, lashes, and walls to help your training and extend presents.

15 to 21 Days Yoga Challenge

Leave on a groundbreaking excursion with this 15 to 21 days yoga challenge. Every day expands upon the last, bit by bit heightening your training and developing your brain body association. Plan to open new degrees of solidarity, adaptability, and inward harmony.

Day 15: Establishing Stream

Morning: Establishing Practice (30 minutes)

Mountain Posture (Tadasana) - 1 moment
Forward Overlap (Uttanasana) - 1 moment
Fighter II (Virabhadrasana II) - 1 moment each side
Triangle Posture (Trikonasana) - 1 moment each side
Youngster's Posture (Balasana) - 2 minutes
Late morning: Pranayama and Contemplation (20 minutes)

Dirga Pranayama (Three-Section Breath)
- 5 minutes
Situated Reflection - 15 minutes
Evening: Supportive Yoga (30 minutes)

Leaning back Bound Point Posture (Supta
Baddha Konasana) - 5 minutes
Recumbent   Wind   (Supta
Matsyendrasana) - 3 minutes each side
Advantages the-Wall Posture (Viparita
Karani) - 5 minutes
Cadaver Posture (Savasana) - 10 minutes
Day 16: Center Strength
Morning: Center Stream (30 minutes)

Boat Posture (Navasana) - 1 moment
Board Posture (Phalakasana) - 1 moment
Side Board (Vasisthasana) - 1 moment
each side
Insect Posture (Salabhasana) - 1 moment
Span Posture (Setu Bandhasana) - 2
minutes

Late morning: Dynamic Recuperation (20 minutes)

Feline Cow Stretch (Marjaryasana-Bitilasana) - 5 minutes
Situated Ahead Twist (Paschimottanasana) - 5 minutes
Situated Wind (Ardha Matsyendrasana) - 5 minutes each side
Kid's Posture (Balasana) - 5 minutes
Evening: Yoga Nidra (30 minutes)

Directed Yoga Nidra Practice - 30 minutes
Day 17: Equilibrium and Adaptability
Morning: Equilibrium and Stretch (30 minutes)

Tree Posture (Vrksasana) - 1 moment each side
Bird Posture (Garudasana) - 1 moment each side
Fighter III (Virabhadrasana III) - 1 moment each side

Half Moon Posture (Ardha Chandrasana) - 1 moment each side

Forward Overlay (Uttanasana) - 2 minutes

Noontime: Yin Yoga (20 minutes)

Mythical serpent Posture (Yin Variety) - 3 minutes each side

Sphinx Posture - 3 minutes

Butterfly Posture (Yin Variety) - 3 minutes

Upheld Fish Posture - 5 minutes

Body Posture (Savasana) - 6 minutes

Evening: Profound Stretch and Unwinding (30 minutes)

Situated Ahead Curve (Paschimottanasana) - 3 minutes

Leaning back Hand-to-Huge Toe Posture (Supta Padangusthasana) - 3 minutes each side

Cheerful Child Posture (Ananda Balasana) - 3 minutes

Leaning back Contort (Supta Matsyendrasana) - 3 minutes each side
Carcass Posture (Savasana) - 10 minutes
Day 18: Strength and Perseverance
Morning: Power Stream (40 minutes)

Sun Greetings (Surya Namaskar) - 5 rounds
Hero I (Virabhadrasana I) - 1 moment each side
Side Board (Vasisthasana) - 1 moment each side
Seat Posture (Utkatasana) - 1 moment
Crow Posture (Bakasana) - 2 minutes
Early afternoon: Dynamic Stream (30 minutes)

Feline Cow Stretch (Marjaryasana-Bitilasana) - 5 minutes
Descending Confronting Canine (Adho Mukha Svanasana) - 5 minutes
Hero II (Virabhadrasana II) Stream - 10 minutes
Camel Posture (Ustrasana) - 5 minutes

Youngster's Posture (Balasana) - 5 minutes
Evening: Profound Unwinding (30 minutes)

Upheld Shoulderstand (Salamba Sarvangasana) - 5 minutes
Fish Posture (Matsyasana) - 3 minutes
Situated Ahead Twist (Paschimottanasana) - 3 minutes
Leaning back Curve (Supta Matsyendrasana) - 5 minutes each side
Cadaver Posture (Savasana) - 10 minutes
Day 19: Backbends and Heart Openers
Morning: Heart Opening Stream (40 minutes)

Cobra Posture (Bhujangasana) - 1 moment
Camel Posture (Ustrasana) - 1 moment each side
Bow Posture (Dhanurasana) - 1 moment
Wheel Posture (Urdhva Dhanurasana) - 1 moment

Fish Posture (Matsyasana) - 2 minutes
Noontime: Pranayama and Reflection (30 minutes)

Kapalabhati (Skull Sparkling Breath) - 5 minutes
Bhramari (Honey bee Breath) - 5 minutes
Anapanasati Contemplation - 20 minutes
Evening: Helpful Yoga (40 minutes)

Upheld Extension Posture (Setu Bandhasana) - 5 minutes
Upheld Fish Posture (Matsyasana) - 5 minutes
Upheld Bound Point Posture (Supta Baddha Konasana) - 5 minutes
Advantages the-Wall Posture (Viparita Karani) - 10 minutes
Directed Unwinding - 15 minutes
Day 20: Reversals and Equilibrium
Morning: Reversal Practice (40 minutes)

Dolphin Posture (Ardha Pincha Mayurasana) - 2 minutes

Headstand (Sirsasana) - 2 minutes

Lower arm Stand (Pincha Mayurasana) - 2 minutes

Handstand (Adho Mukha Vrksasana) - 2 minutes

Upheld Shoulderstand (Salamba Sarvangasana) - 5 minutes

Carcass Posture (Savasana) - 5 minutes

Early afternoon: Center and Solidness (30 minutes)

Boat Posture (Navasana) - 3 minutes

Board Posture (Phalakasana) - 3 minutes

Side Board (Vasisthasana) - 2 minutes each side

Insect Posture (Salabhasana) - 3 minutes

Span Posture (Setu Bandhasana) - 3 minutes

Cadaver Posture (Savasana) - 5 minutes

Evening: Delicate Stretch and Unwinding (40 minutes)

Youngster's Posture (Balasana) - 5 minutes

Leaning back Bound Point Posture (Supta Baddha Konasana) - 5 minutes
Recumbent Wind (Supta Matsyendrasana) - 5 minutes each side
Situated Ahead Curve (Paschimottanasana) - 5 minutes
Body Posture (Savasana) - 20 minutes
Day 21: Reflection and Festivity
Morning: Festivity Stream (45 minutes)

Sun Greetings (Surya Namaskar) - 5 rounds
Champion Stream (Virabhadrasana I, II, III) - 3 minutes each side
Backbend Grouping (Cobra, Camel, Wheel) - 3 minutes each
Adjusting Stances (Tree, Hawk, Half Moon) - 2 minutes each side
Reversal Practice (Headstand, Handstand) - 3 minutes each
Last Unwinding - 5 minutes
Early afternoon: Appreciation Practice (30 minutes)

Journaling - Consider your excursion and offer thanks for your training.

Directed Perception - Imagine your future yoga excursion and set expectations.

Evening: Shutting Function (an hour)

Helpful Yoga - Delicate stretches to deliver strain.

Contemplation and Shutting Circle - Consider your accomplishments and set expectations for what's to come.

Sharing Circle - Offer bits of knowledge and encounters with individual specialists.

Shutting Contemplation - Seal your training with appreciation and love.

Congrats on finishing the 21-day yoga challenge! Pause for a minute to respect yourself for your responsibility and commitment to your training. May you convey the harmony, strength, and shrewdness acquired from these previous days into the following period of your excursion. Namaste.

Conclusion

In the climax of this yoga venture, you've navigated through long periods of careful development, profound breathing, and significant self-revelation. Every day carried new difficulties to survive, new qualities to reveal, and new profundities of inward harmony to investigate. As you consider your encounters, you might find that the genuine substance of yoga reaches out a long ways past the actual stances; it lives in the association between psyche, body, and soul.

Through this training, you've developed flexibility, persistence, and sympathy, both on and off the mat. You've figured out how to pay attention to the murmurs of your body, to embrace the cadence of your breath, and to calm the jabber of your psyche. In snapshots of tranquility, you've found the limitlessness of your own being — the endless potential that lives inside you.

As you finish up this excursion, recollect that yoga isn't just a progression of stances or groupings; it is a lifestyle — a continuous investigation of mindfulness and self-revelation. Whether you keep on rehearsing yoga day to day or discontinuously, may you convey the examples learned and the changes experienced with you generally.

As you step off the mat and into the world, may you move with beauty, talk with generosity, and live with goal. Furthermore, may the light that sparkles inside you enlighten the way forward, directing you towards more prominent love, euphoria, and satisfaction.

Breathe in profoundly, breathe out completely, and embrace the limitless conceivable outcomes that anticipate. The excursion of yoga is endless, and with each step in the right direction, you draw nearer to the genuine quintessence of your being.

Namaste.

<u>REQUESTING TO LEAVE A REVIEW</u>

www.ingramcontent.com/pod-product-compliance
Lightning Source LLC
Chambersburg PA
CBHW071042250726

48653CB00005B/1959